The Physician's Guide to
Mother Goose

ISBN 978-1-950034-82-6 (Paperback)
The Physician's Guide to Mother Goose
Copyright © 2019 by TK Denmark, MD

Yorkshire Publishing
4613 E. 91st St,
Tulsa, OK 74137
www. YorkshirePublishing. com
918. 394. 2665

Printed in the USA

The Physician's Guide to
Mother Goose

TK Denmark, MD

T U L S A

Contents

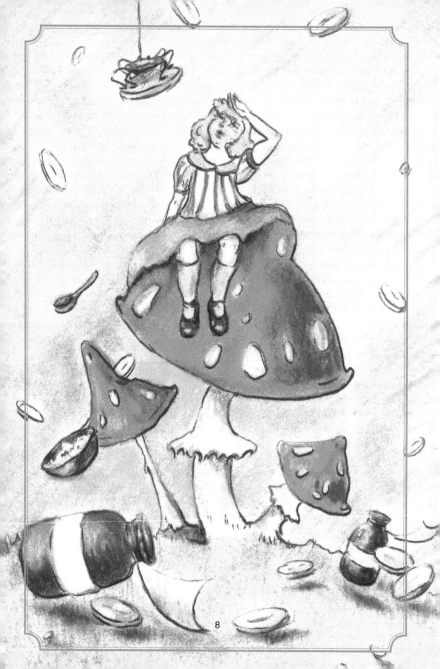

Little Miss Muffet

Little Miss Muffet
Sat on a tuffet,
Eating her curds and whey;
Along came a spider,
Who sat down beside her,
And frightened Miss Muffet away.
And then Miss Muffet developed an abscess which she
swore was a spider bite, and "doctor can you tell me
what kind of spider it was from the color of the pus?"
and "I'm allergic to every pain medication EXCEPT
that one that starts with D..Duh..Duh.. oh, I can never
remember...."

ICD-10:

- 682.5
  (cutaneous abscess of buttock)

- T63.30
  (toxic effect of unspecified spider venom)

- F 15.151
  (other stimulant abuse with stimulant-induced
  psychotic disorder with hallucinations)

Jack and Jill

Jack and Jill went up the hill
To fetch a pail of water;
Jack fell down and broke his crown,
and Jill came tumbling after.
And Jill called 911 and stayed right in Jack's grill
yelling "Don't go to the light Jack!" repeatedly, thereby
saving his life.

ICD-10:

- *S06.OXOA*
  (concussion without loss of consciousness, initial encounter)

- *S01.01XA*
  (laceration without foreign body of scalp, initial encounter)

- *W17.81XA*
  (fall down embankment (hill), initial encounter)

- *Z72.810*
  (truancy, childhood from school)

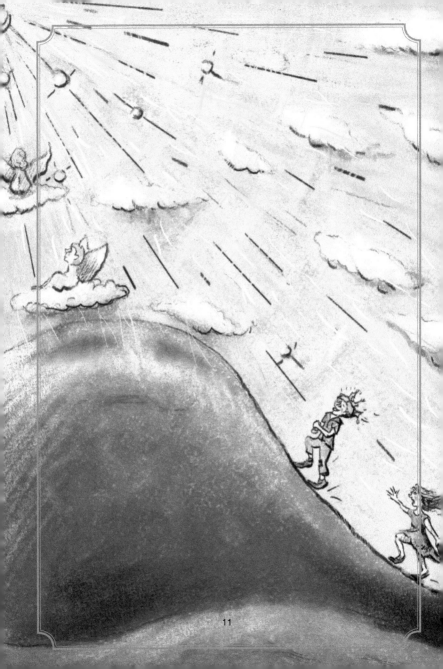

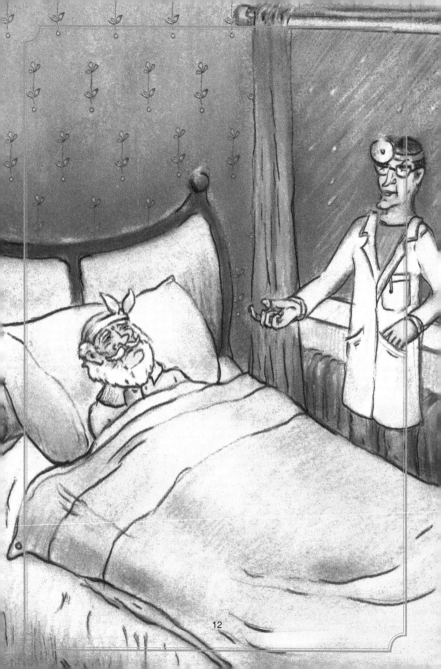

It's Raining, It's Pouring

It's raining, it's pouring,
   The old man's snoring.
He got into bed
   And bumped his head
And couldn't get up in the morning.
And developed post-concussive symptoms that lasted
for months with his primary care physician repeatedly
sending him to the ER to get a CT scan for his concus-
sion symptoms

ICD-10:

- S06.0X4S
  *(concussion with loss of consciousness
  of 6 hours to 24 hours, sequela)*

- G47.33
  (obstructive sleep apnea)

- T59.7X1S
  *(toxic effect of carbon dioxide, accidental
  (unintentional), sequela)*

Hey, Diddle, Diddle

Hey, diddle, diddle,
The cat and the fiddle,
The cow jumped over the moon;
The little dog laughed
To see such sport,
And the dish ran away with the spoon.
But following reentry into the atmosphere, the cow
landed on a passenger on a ship causing injury

ICD-10:

- *W55.22XA*
  (struck by cow, initial encounter)

- *W20.8XXA*
  *(other cause of strike by thrown, projected
  or falling object, initial encounter)*

- *V93.41XA*
  *(struck by falling object on passenger
  ship, initial encounter)*

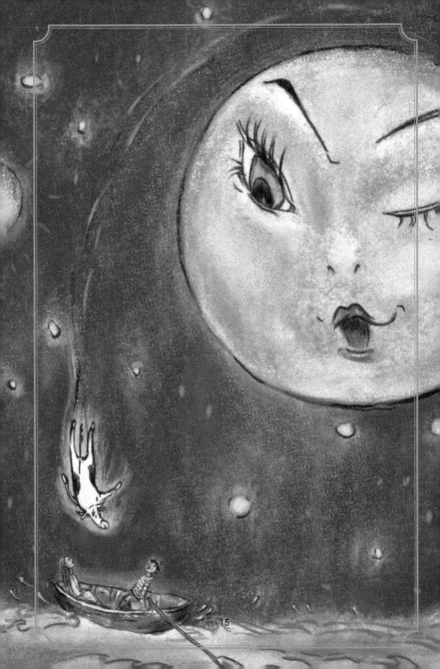

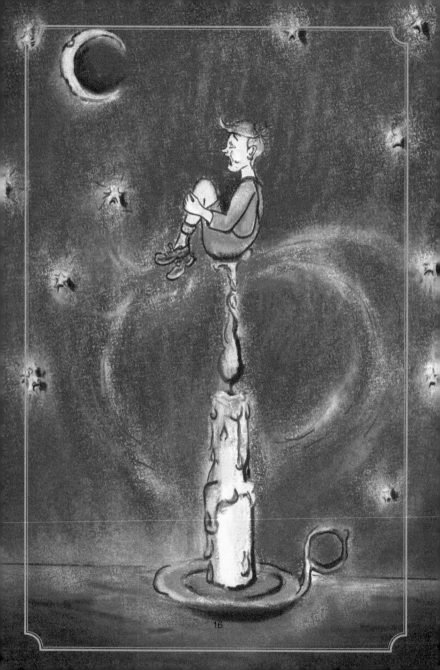

Jack Be Nimble

Jack be nimble,
Jack be quick,
Jack jump over
The candlestick.
But misjudged and slipped and "just fell right on the
candlestick while naked doc, I swear...."

ICD-10:

- T18.5XXA
  (foreign body in anus and rectum, initial encounter)

- T21.25XA
  (burn of second decree of buttock, initial encounter)

Baa, Baa, Black Sheep

Baa, baa, black sheep
Have you any wool?
Yes sir, yes sir, three bags full.
One for the master (who contracted Orf virus),
And one for the dame (who developed Q fever),
And one for the little boy (who acquired Brucellosis)
Who lives down the lane.

ICD-10:

- B08.02
  (Orf disease)

- A78
  (Q fever)

- A23.9
  (Brucellosis)

- FYI:
  All are infections from contact with sheep or wool

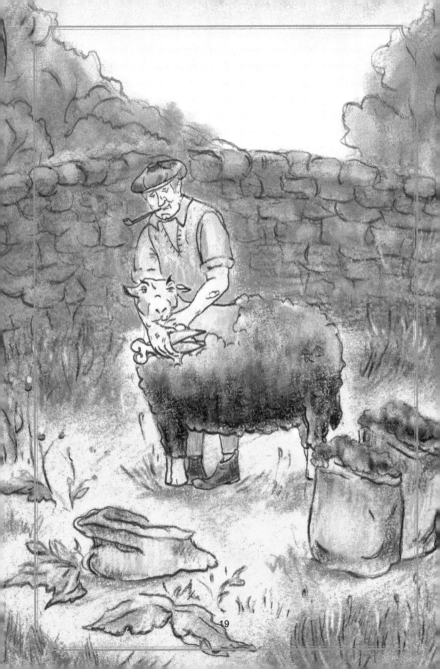

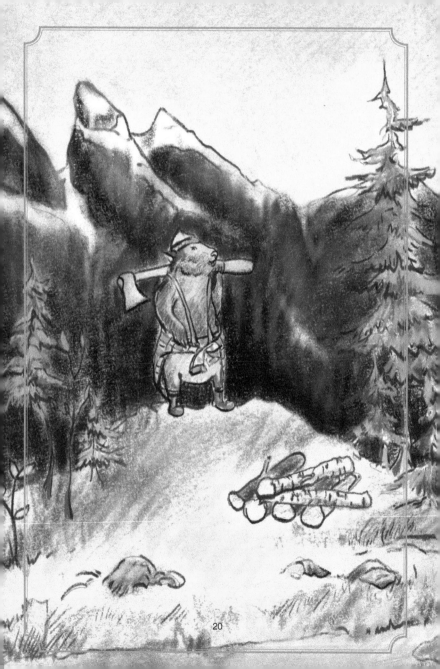

How Much Wood Could a Woodchuck Chuck?

How much wood could a woodchuck chuck
If a woodchuck could chuck wood?
As much wood as a woodchuck could chuck,
If a woodchuck could chuck wood.
Without injuring his lower back, since he's a competitive
little weekend warrior bastard.

ICD-10:

- *S39.012A*
  *(strain of muscle, fascia and tendon of
  lower back, initial encounter)*

Hickory, Dickory, Dock

Hickory, dickory, dock,
The mouse ran up the clock;
The clock struck one,
The mouse went down,
Hickory, dickory, dock.
And ran into the mistress of the house, causing her to
"done fall out".

ICD-10:

- R55
  (vasovagal syncope)

- W53.09
  (accidental contact with mouse)

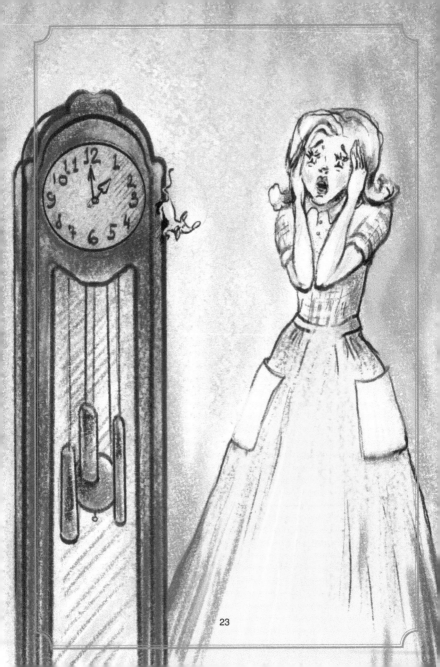

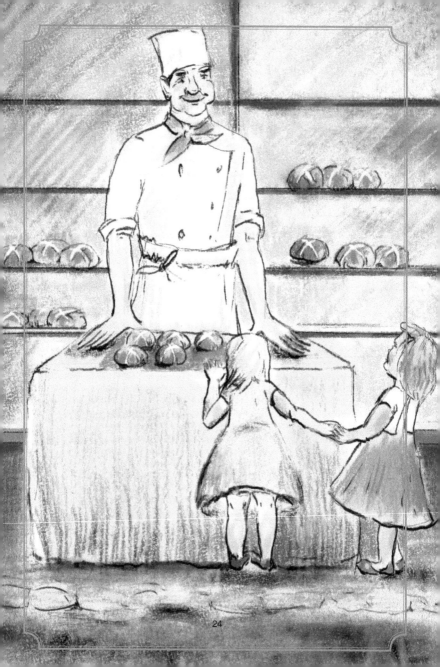

Hot Cross Buns!

Hot-cross buns!
Hot-cross buns!
One a penny, two a penny,
Hot-cross buns!
~~If you have no daughters,~~
~~Give them to your sons,~~
If your daughters eating keto,
Give them to your sons,
One a penny, two a penny,
Hot-cross buns!

ICD-10:

- E16.2
  (hypoglycemia, unspecified)

- Z71.3
  (dietary counseling and surveillance)

Humpty Dumpty

Humpty Dumpty sat on a wall,
Humpty Dumpty had a great fall;
All the king's horses and all the king's men
Couldn't put Humpty together again.
Which is why horses are no longer used for medicinal
and healing activities...

ICD-10:

- *W19.XXXA*
  (accident due to mechanical fall without
  injury, initial encounter)

- *M53.2X1*
  (spinal instabilities, occipito-atlanto-axial region)

- *T79.9XXa*
  (unspecified early complication of
  trauma, initial encounter)

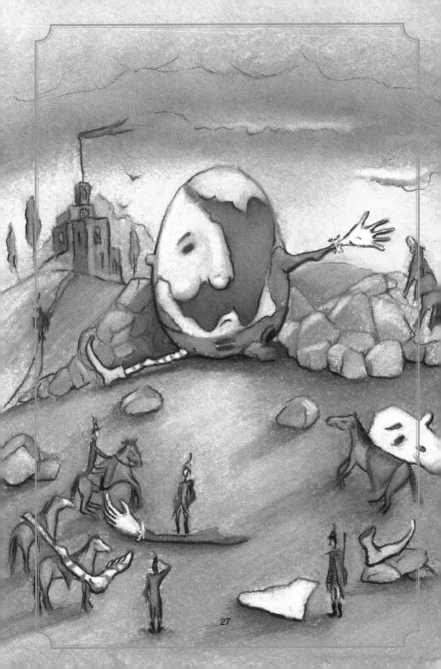

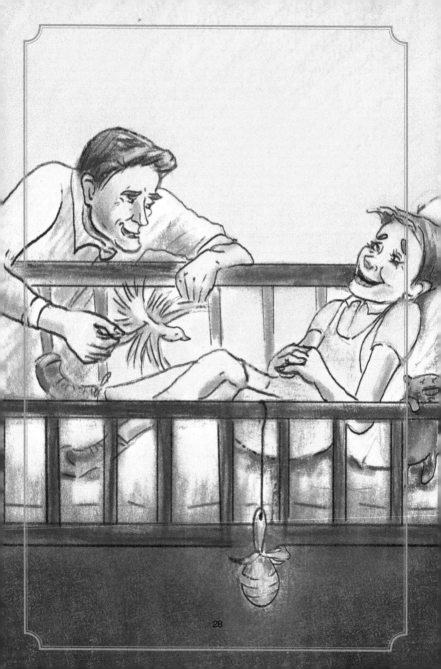

Hush Little Baby

Hush little baby, don't say a word,
Papa's gonna buy you a mockingbird.

And if that mockingbird won't sing,
Papa's gonna buy you a diamond ring.
Because you're a spoiled little baby destined to be a
snowflake millennial...

ICD-10:

- Z73.4
  (inadequate social skills, not elsewhere classified)

- Z62.1
  (overprotection, child by parent)

Ladybird, Ladybird

Ladybird, ladybird,
Fly away home,
Your house is on fire
And your children all gone;
All except one
And that's little Ann,
And she has crept under
The warming pan.
Where stop drop and roll is not working out very well
for her....

ICD-10:

- Y07.12
  (biological mother, perpetrator of maltreatment and neglect)

- Z62.0
  (lack of parental supervision or control of child)

- T21.23
  (burn of second degree of upper back)

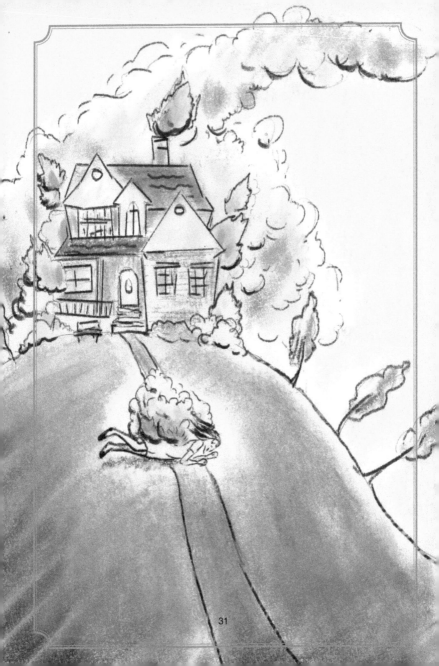

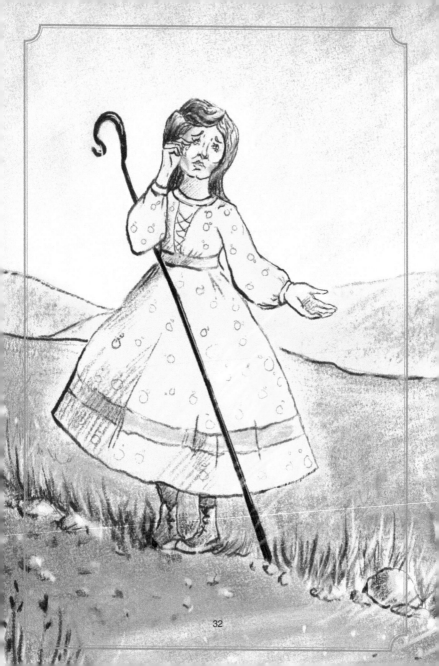

Little Bo-Peep

Little Bo-Peep has lost her sheep,
And can't tell where to find them;
Leave them alone, and they'll come home,
Bringing their tails behind them.
But without livelihood, Bo-Peep couldn't pay
her mortgage,
So she is now panhandling at the highway offramp

ICD-10:

- Z59.0
  (homelessness)

- Z63.5
  (disruption of family due to separation)

- Z59.5
  (extreme poverty NEC)

Little Boy Blue

Little boy blue,
Come blow your horn,
The sheep's in the meadow,
The cow's in the corn.
But where is the boy
Who looks after the sheep?
He's under a haystack,
Fast asleep. (although he is actually cyanotic, but
revived with resuscitative efforts...)

ICD-10:

- G47.419
  (narcolepsy without cataplexy)

- T71.191A
  (asphyxiation due to mechanical threat to breathing due to other causes, accidental)… the haystack

- G47.19
  (daytime hypersomnia)

- R23.9
  (cyanosis)

- I46.8
  (Cardiac arrest due to specified condition NEC)

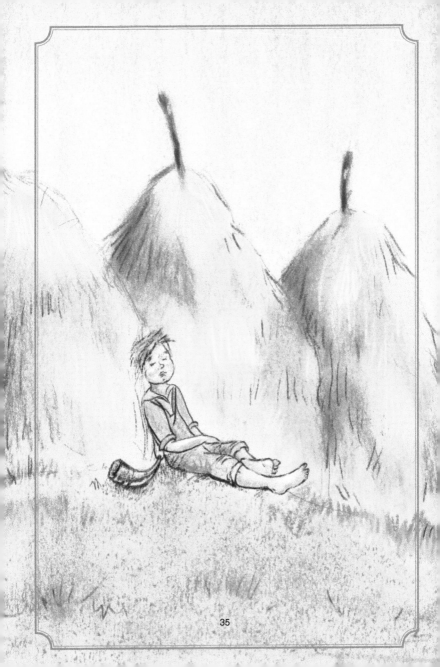

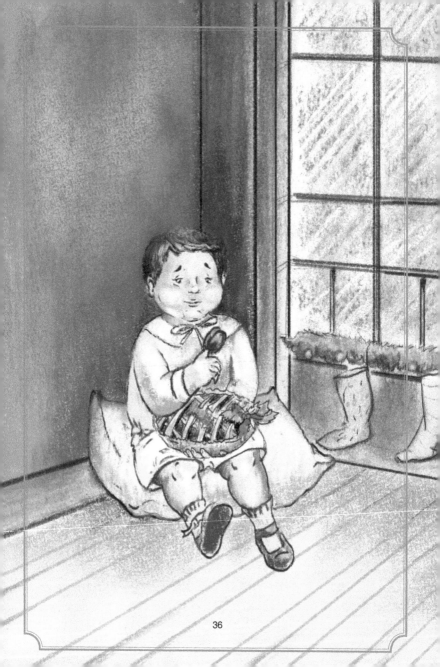

Little Jack Horner

Plump Jack Horner
Sat in the corner,
Eating a Christmas pie;
He put in his thumb,
And pulled out a plum,
And said, "What a good boy am I!"
Followed by "Holy crap! My back! I threw my back out!"

ICD-10:

- F60.81
  (narcissistic personality disorder)

- Z72.810
  (child antisocial behavior)

- Z73.4
  (inadequate social skills, not elsewhere classified)

- E66.01
  (Mobid (severe) obesity due to excess calories)

- M62.830
  (Muscle spasm of back)

Mary, Mary, Quite Contrary

Mary, Mary, quite contrary
How does your garden grow?
With silver bells and cockleshells
And UV grow-lights over the medicinal marijuana

ICD-10:

- *F91.3*
  (oppositional defiance conduct disorder of childhood)

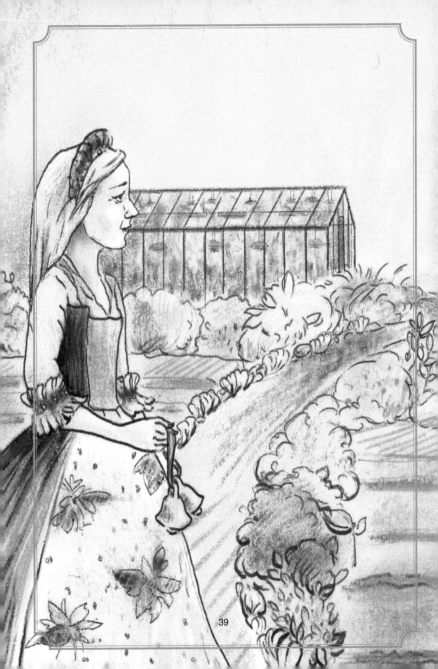

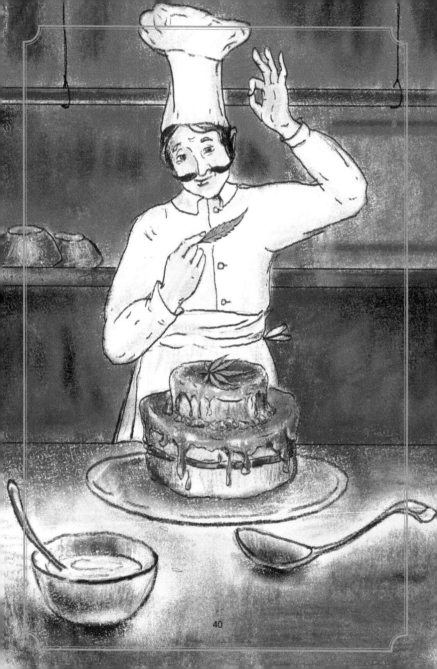

Pat-A-Cake, Pat-A-Cake

Pat-a-cake, pat-a-cake, baker's man,
Bake me a cake, as fast as you can;
Pat it, prick it, and mark it with B,
~~Put it in the oven for baby and me.~~
Put some Mary J in it for baby and me.

ICD-10:

- F12.122
  *(Cannabis abuse with intoxication
  and perceptual disturbance)*

- F12.280
  *(cannabis dependence with cannabis-
  induced anxiety disorder)*

Pease Porridge Hot

Pease porridge hot,
Pease porridge cold,
Pease porridge in the pot
Nine days old.

ICD-10:

- T62.91XA
  (toxic effect of unspecified noxious substance eaten as food, accidental (unintentional), initial encounter)

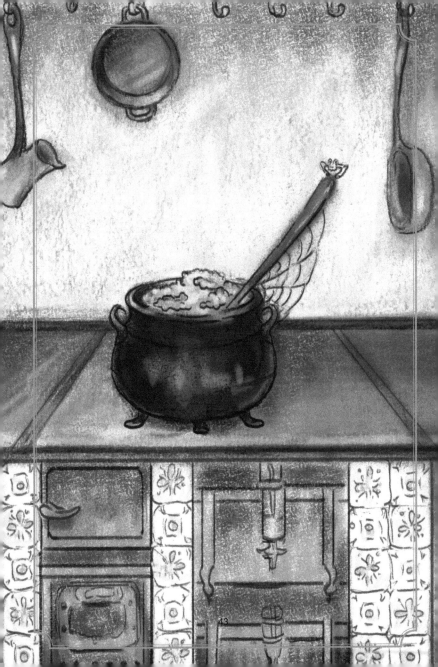

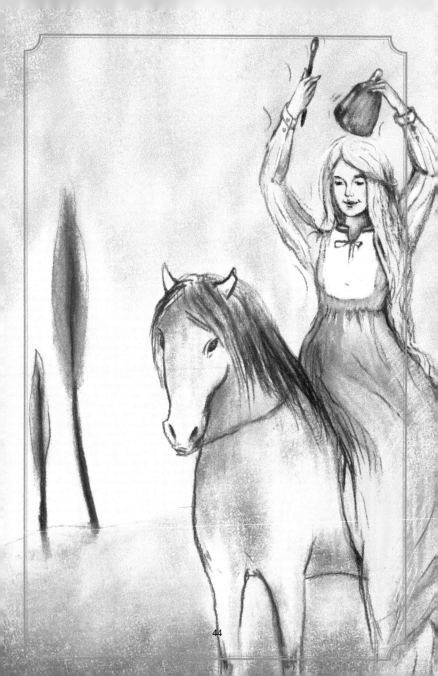

Ride a Cockhorse to Banbury Cross

Ride a cockhorse to Banbury Cross,
To see a fine lady upon a white horse;
Rings on her fingers and bells on her toes,
~~She shall have music wherever she goes.~~
She'll have more cowbell wherever she goes.

ICD-10:

- H83.3X3
  (noise effects on inner ear, bilateral)

Ring Around the Rosy

Ring around the rosy,
Pocket full of posy,
Ashes!   Ashes!
We all fall down!

ICD-10:

- *W01.0XXA*
  (fall on same level from slipping, tripping and stumbling without subsequent striking against object, initial encounter)

- *T17.500A*
  (unspecified foreign body in bronchus causing asphyxiation, initial encounter)

- *A20.2*
  (pneumonic plague)

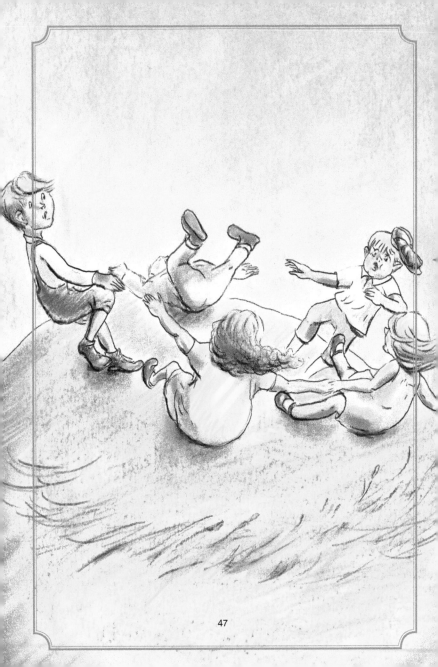

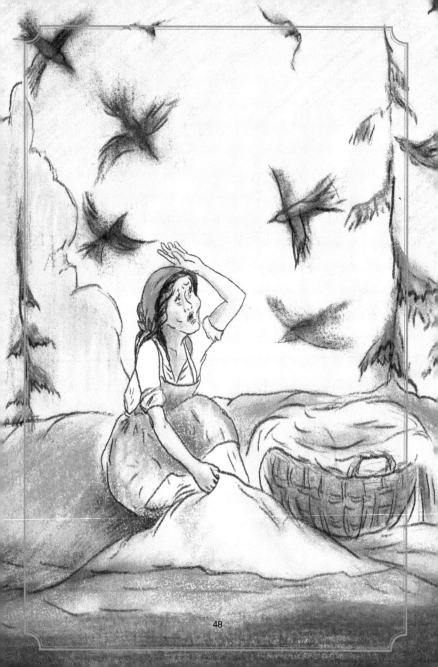

Sing a Song of Sixpence

Sing a song of sixpence,
A pocket full of rye,
Four and twenty blackbirds
Baked in a pie.

When the pie was opened
The birds began to sing—
Wasn't that a dainty dish
To set before the king?

The king was in the
counting-house

Counting out his money,
The queen was in the
parlor
Eating bread and honey.

The maid was in the
garden
Hanging out the clothes.
Along came a blackbird
And snipped off her nose.

ICD-10:

- *W61.91*
  (bitten by other, birds)

- *S08.811A*
  *(Complete traumatic amputation
  of nose, initial encounter)*

There Was a Crooked Man

There was a crooked man, and he walked a crooked mile,
He found a crooked sixpence against a crooked stile;
He bought a crooked cat which caught a crooked mouse,
And they all lived inebriated together in a little crooked house.

ICD-10:

- M41.20
  (other idiopathic scoliosis, site unspecified)

- F10.229
  (alcohol dependence with intoxication, unspecified)

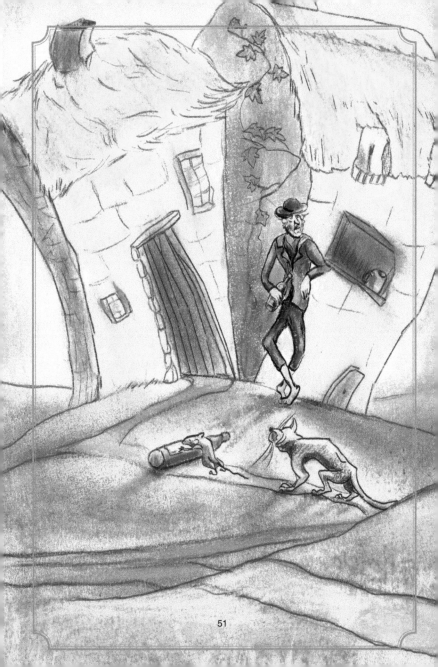

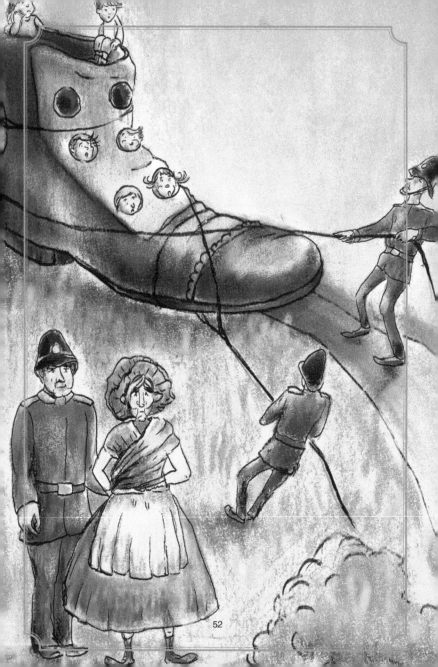

The Old Woman Who Lived in a Shoe

There was an old woman who lived in a shoe.
She had so many children, she didn't know what to do.
She gave them some broth without any bread;
And whipped them all soundly and put them to bed
And DHS removed them from her custody and placed
them all in foster care.

ICD-10:

- T38.4X6
  (Underdosing of oral contraceptives (baby))

- T76.02XA
  (child neglect or abandonment,
  suspected, initial encounter)

- Z59.1
  (lack of adequate housing)

- Z02.81
  (encounter for paternity testing)

This Little Piggy

This little piggy went to market,
This little piggy stayed home,
This little piggy had roast beef,
This little piggy had none.
This little piggy went ...
Running away from his vaccine injections making him a
threat to society, so
They made him bacon

ICD-10:

- *R39.81*
  (functional urinary incontinence)

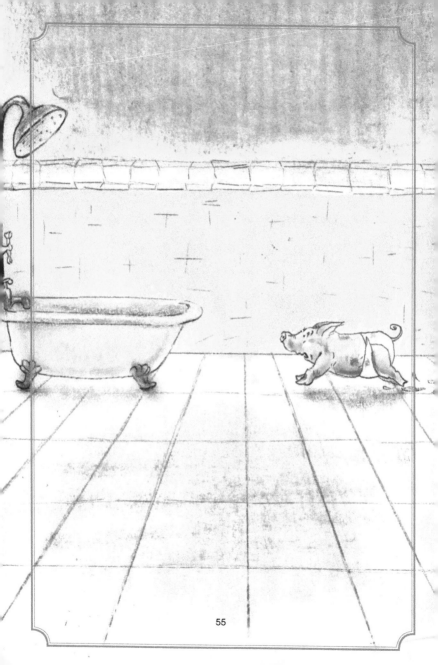

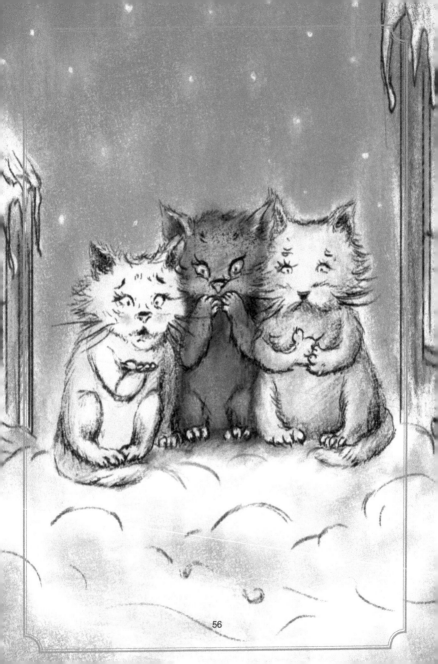

Three Little Kitten

The three little kittens, they lost their mittens,
And they began to cry,
"Oh, mother dear, we sadly fear,
That we have lost our mittens."
"What! Lost your mittens, you naughty kittens!
Then you shall have no pie."
"Meow, meow, meow."
"Then you shall have no pie,
And your paws will be very cold."

ICD-10:

- I73.00
  (Raynaud's syndrome)

- T74.02Xa
  (child victim of nutritional neglect)

- R68.12
  (fussy baby)

Yankee Doodle

Yankee Doodle went to town,
A-riding on a pony;
Stuck a feather in his hat
And called it macaroni.

ICD-10:

- R48.8
  (anomia)

- F22.59
  (Delusional disorder, grandiose type, first
  episode, currently in acute episode)

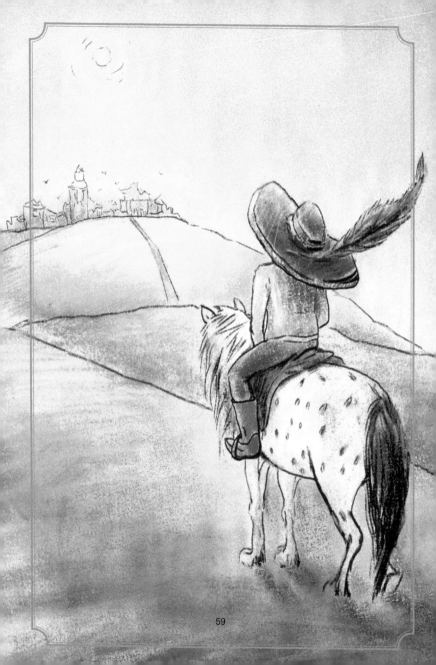

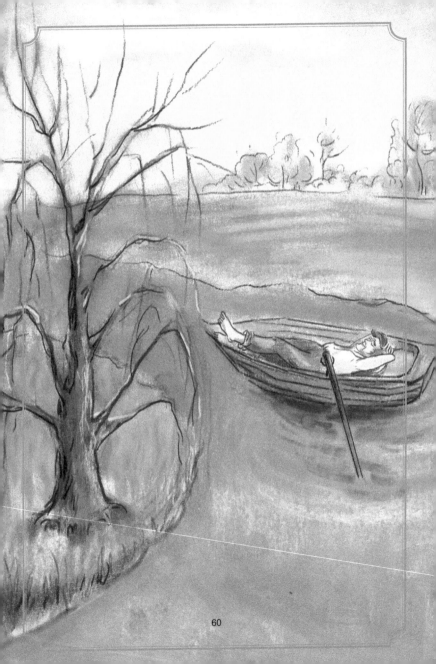

Row, Row, Row Your Boat

Row, row, row your boat
Gently down the stream.
Merrily, merrily, merrily, merrily,
Life is but a dream

ICD-10:

- F16.12
  (Hallucinogen abuse with intoxication)

- V91.82XA
  *(Other injury due to other accident,
  fishing boat, initial encounter)*

Rock-a-Bye Baby

Rock-a-bye baby, on the treetops,
When the wind blows, the cradle will rock,
When the bough breaks, the cradle will fall
And down will come baby, cradle and all.

ICD-10:

- W14
  (Fall from tree, initial encounter)

- T74.92XA
  (Unspecified child maltreatment,
  confirmed, initial encounter)

- Z62.0
  (Inadequate parental supervision and control)

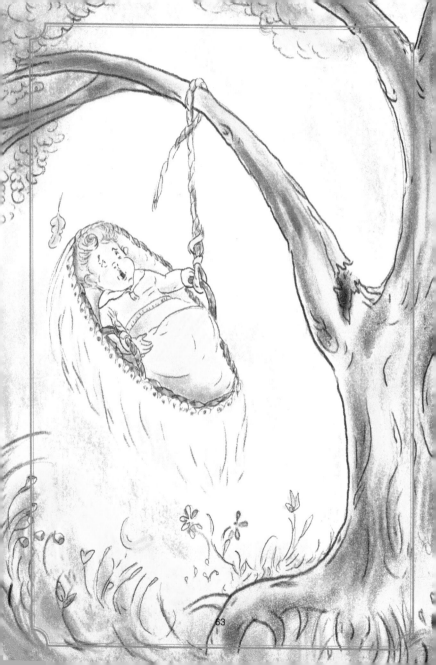

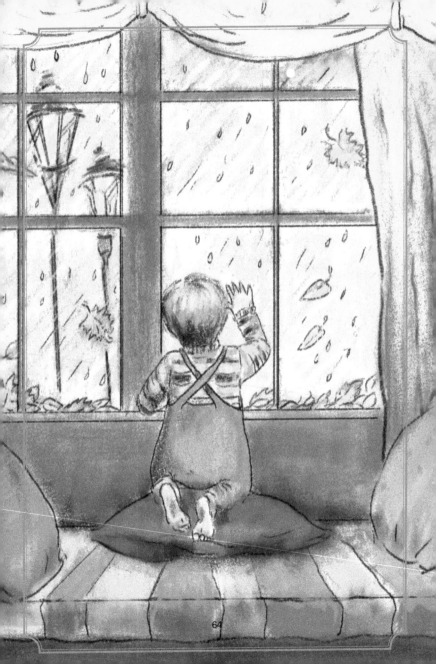

Rain, Rain Go Away

Rain, rain go away
Come again another day.
Since you make my SAD flair when you're gray.

ICD-10:

- F33.859
  (Seasonal affective disorder)

Pop! Goes The Weasel

All around the Mulberry bush,
The monkey chased the weasel.
The monkey stopped to pull up his sock,
Pop! Goes the weasel.
And DOWN goes the monkey....

ICD-10:

- *R06.89*
  (Other abnormalities of breathing,
  breath-holding (spells))

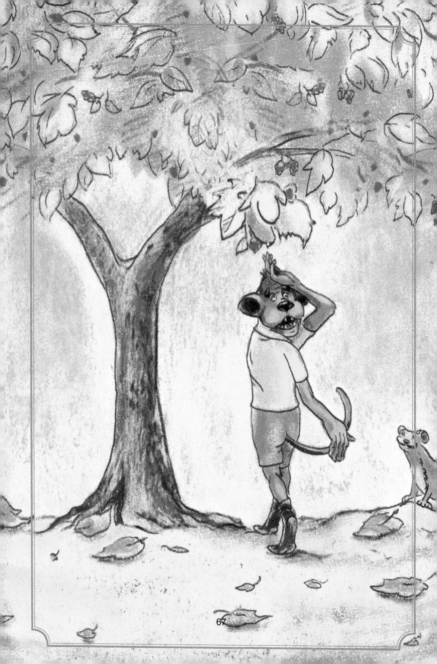

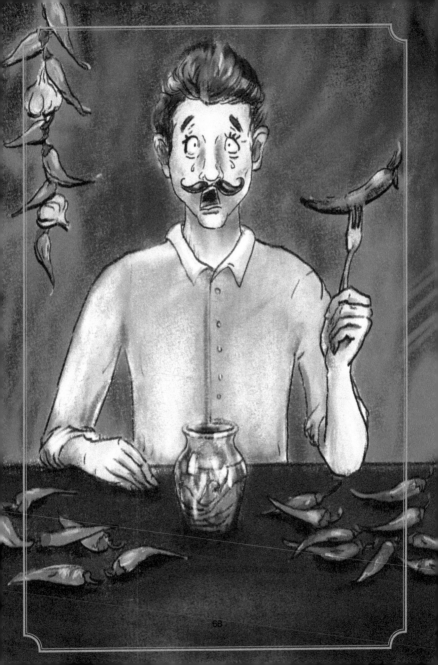

Peter Piper Picked A Peck of Pickled Peppers

Peter Piper picked a peck of pickled peppers,
A peck of pickled peppers Peter Piper picked;
If Peter Piper picked a peck of pickled peppers,
Where's the peck of pickled peppers Peter Piper picked?

ICD-10:

- *T28.0XXA*
  (Burn of mouth and pharynx, initial encounter)

Peter, Peter Pumpkin Eater

Peter, Peter pumpkin eater,
Had a wife but couldn't keep her;
He put her in a pumpkin shell
And there he kept her very well.

ICD-10:

- T74.01XA
  *(Adult neglect or abandonment,
  confirmed, initial encounter)*

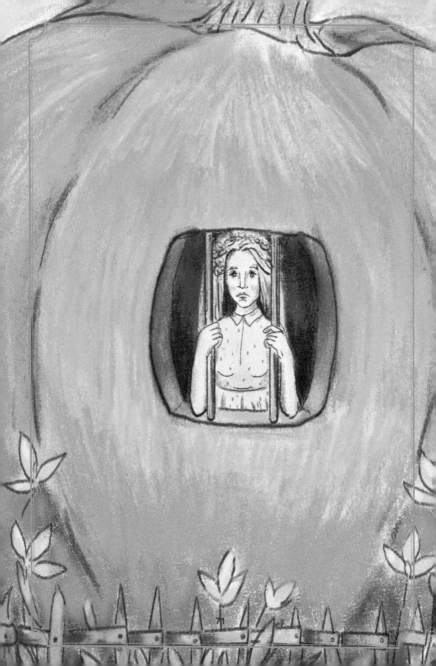

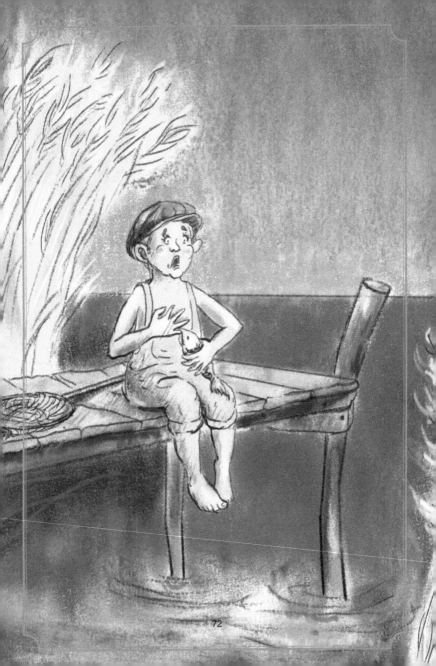

1, 2, 3, 4, 5...
Once I Caught A Fish Alive!

One, two, three, four, five,
Once I caught a fish alive,
Six, seven, eight, nine, ten,
Then I let it go again.
Why did you let it go?
Because it bit my finger so.
Which finger did it bite?
This little finger on my right.

ICD-10:

- *W56.51XA*
  (Fish bite wound, initial encounter)

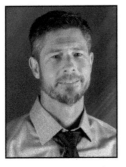

T. Kent Denmark knew it was important to grow up, but how to retain youthful vigor and silliness while practicing medicine? By choosing pediatrics, of course! And not just any field of pediatrics, but pediatric emergency medicine where the ability to charm, tease or cajole pint sized patients is essential. But what he discovered is that there is an even greater silliness at work – serious grownups refer to it as ICD 10, and they wear suits and rest their chins in their hands while nodding and having very serious expressions. But how can you have a serious expression on your face while creating a code (V93.D) for "Burn due to water-skis on fire, subsequent encounter". So, with a (clean version) nod to Andrew Dice Clay, he decided to provide medical billing codes for Mother Goose.